Homemade Remedies

Medicines My Momma Made

BY

Rachael Rayner

License Notes

No part of this Book can be reproduced in any form or by any means including print, electronic, scanning or photocopying unless prior permission is granted by the author.

All ideas, suggestions and guidelines mentioned here are written for informative purposes. While the author has taken every possible step to ensure accuracy, all readers are advised to follow information at their own risk. The author cannot be held responsible for personal and/or commercial damages in case of misinterpreting and misunderstanding any part of this Book

Table of Contents

Introduction

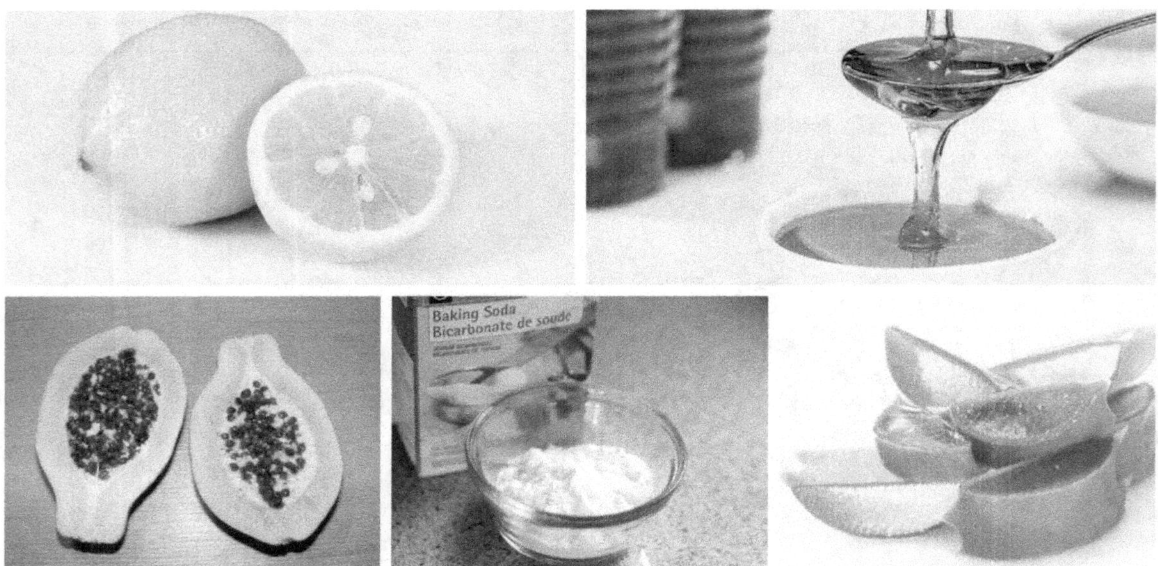

We all dream of going back in time when all medicines were pretty much homemade; herbs and spices were always used to make medicines or creams. Sore throat, colds, and flu were treated with liquid concoctions made from the herb garden. You could also make creams and salves to help with burns, aches, or sores.

There are simple treatments to prepare in your home, distributed by you. Some of these can be passed down through the family. The pioneers and native Americans used all types of items in their homemade remedies. Remedies can be made to treat sleep, cough, cold, earache, or hair loss.

People like the idea of using home items to make anything that doesn't cost an arm and a leg. We know how much medicines and doctor visits cost.

We have learned to make soaps and lotions; now we need to learn how to use Mother Nature's goodness and make some homemade items. It can range from tinctures to teas. There are so many choices to make with herbs and household items.

Spices can be mixed with vinegar to make a cough syrup. Fruit pulp can be used to calm arthritis, and cucumbers can be placed over eyes when a headache arrives. The mixtures can be endless. You can also save money. Be sure and try some.

Medicinal Homemade Recipes

Salt Sock Earache Home Remedy

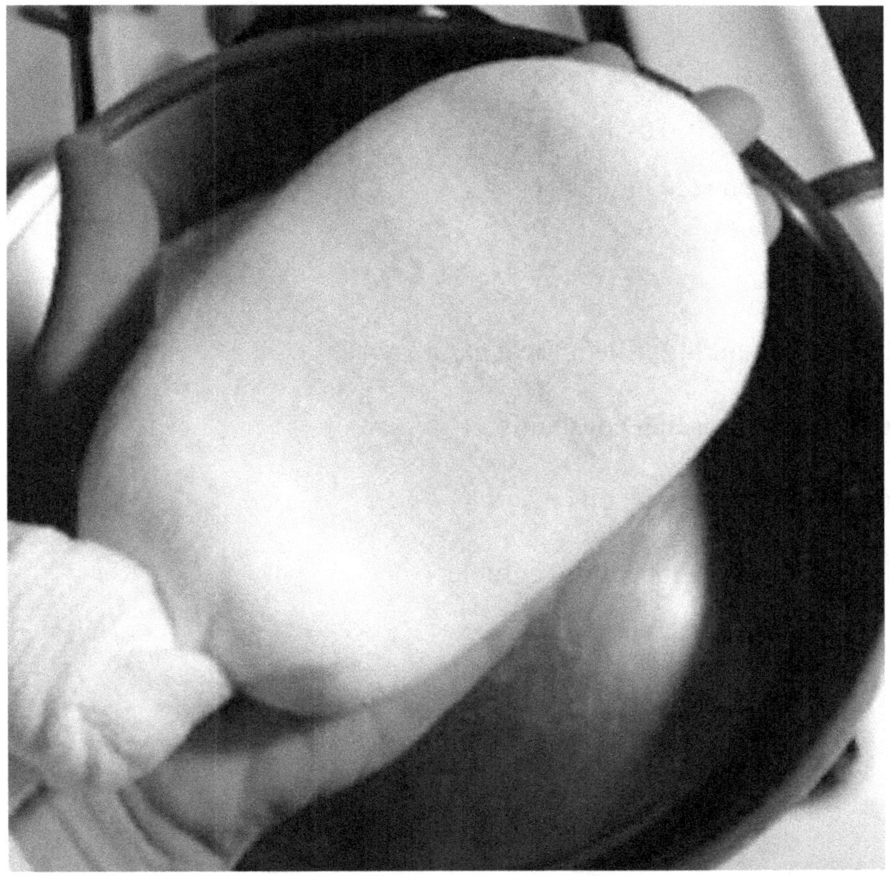

Earaches can be very painful. When one hits, relief is all we want. The ease of making this sock is as simple as finding an old sock, then follow the directions.

Prep Time: 10 minutes

Yields: 1 sock

Ingredients:

- White Sock, 1
- Skillet, med.
- Coarse Sea Salt, ¾ of the sock
- Basil Essential Oil, 10 drops
- Lavender Seasoned Oil, 8 drops

Directions:

1. Pour salt into sock until ¾ filled. Tie a good knot.

2. Heat sock in skillet, turning constantly.

3. Spread drops of the essential oils over the sock.

4. Use on ear until heat is gone. It is reusable.

Homemade Ear Wax Removal Recipe

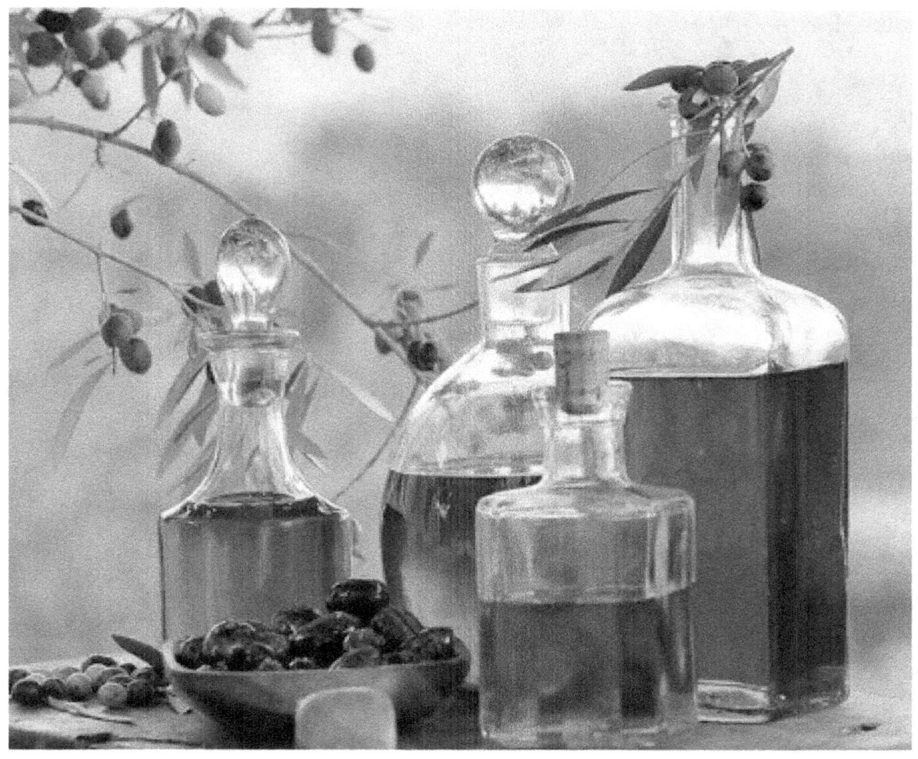

Wax can build up fast in an ear. You can use over-the-counter ear drops or go to see the doctor and get the wax professionally removed. However, ear drops can be made at home and a lot cheaper. Try this!

Prep Time: 20 minutes

Yields: 1 bottle

Ingredients:

- Saline Solution, 1 Tbs.
- Water, 1 cup

Directions:

1. Combine the saline solution and water.

2. Put several drops in the ears.

3. Hold head at an angle to keep the drops in for several minutes.

4. Then turn head and let the mixture drain out.

You can also use any of the following to remove wax:

- Vinegar and rubbing alcohol
- Olive Oil
- Glycerin
- Hydrogen Peroxide
- Paraffin Oil

Homemade Cough Syrup Recipe

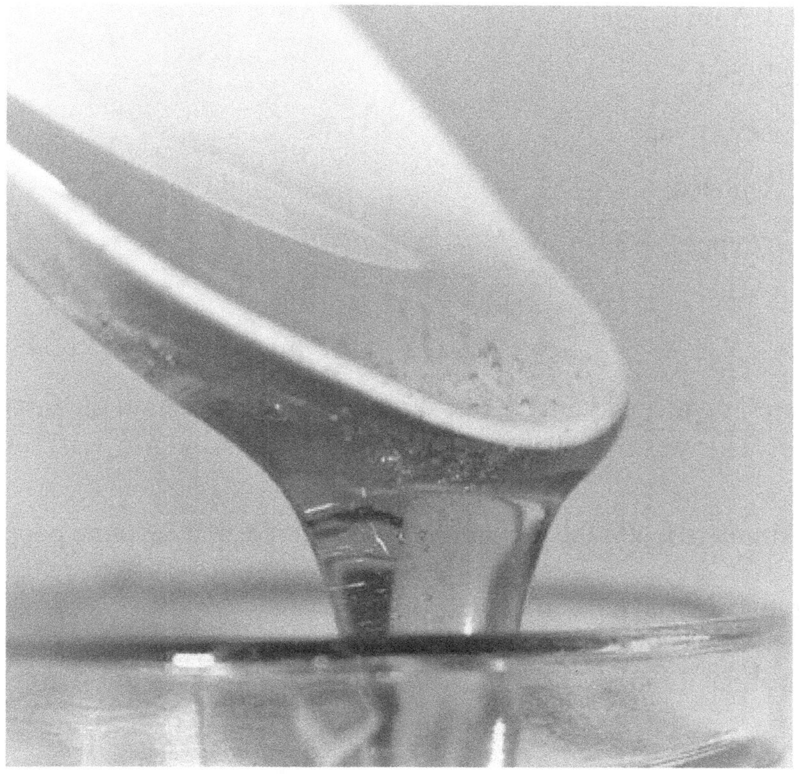

You should always have cough syrup on hand. When cold weather starts and grandchildren spend time with you, you need to have this. This homemade cough works wonders for the young and the old.

Prep Time: 20 minutes

Yields: 2 cups

Ingredients:

- Water, 2 cups
- Thyme, 8 fresh sprigs
- Ginger, ¼ cup
- Raw Honey, 1 cup
- Lemon, 1 juiced
- Cayenne Pepper, 1/8 tsp.

Directions:

1. Combine water, thyme, and ginger and simmer on the stove until the mixture is reduced to half.

2. Once it has simmered, add the raw honey, lemon juice, and cayenne pepper.

3. Strain to remove debris, pour in jar and store.

4. Shelf time is about 2 months.

Homemade Decongestant Tablets for Shower

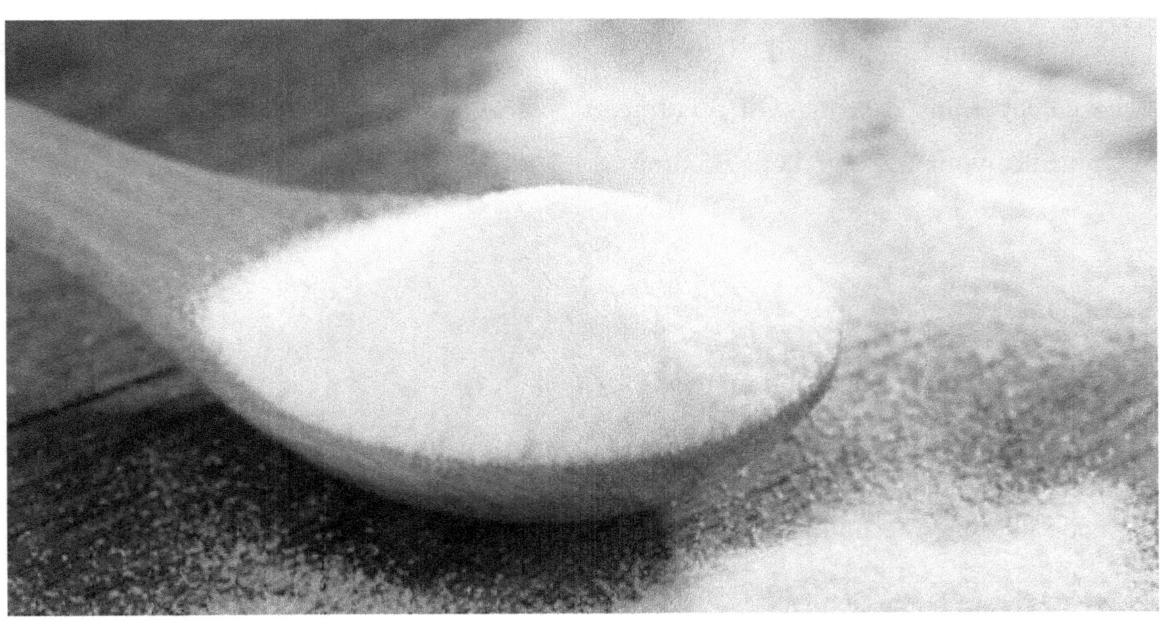

Steam from a shower can help open airways for asthmatics. These shower tablets help to open your sinuses. Take your shower and open your sinuses at the same time.

Prep Time: 30 minutes

Yields: 10 Tablets

Ingredients:

- Baking Soda, 1 cup
- Citric Acid, ½ cup
- Cornstarch, ¼ cup
- Camphor Essential Oil, 50 drops
- Peppermint Essential Oil, 35 drops
- Eucalyptus Essential Oil, 35 drops
- Water, 2 tsp.

Directions:

1. Combine all ingredients and mix well.

2. Line a muffin tin with cupcake liners.

3. Scoop mixture in each liner.

4. Set aside and let harden.

5. Store in closed packaging until using.

Phlegm Removal Home Remedy

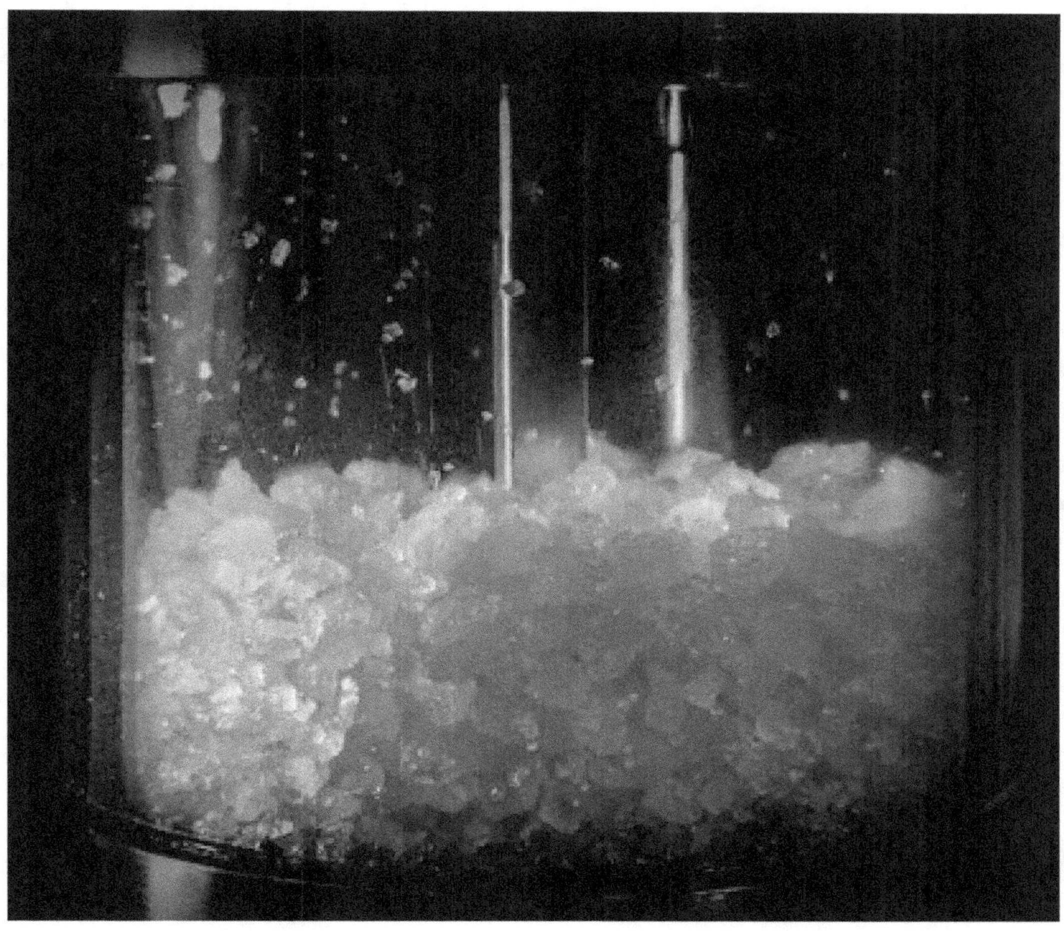

We have all had colds where the phlegm keeps building up. We cough and cough without any results of coughing it up. These home concoctions will help.

Prep Time: 15 minutes

Yields: 1 glass

Ingredients:

- Turmeric, 1 tsp.
- Salt, ½ tsp
- Water, 1 Glass

Directions:

1. Combine all ingredients together and mix well.

2. Use as a gargle one to two times a day until gone.

3. It will help destroy bacteria.

Ginger Tea Mucus Remover Home Remedy

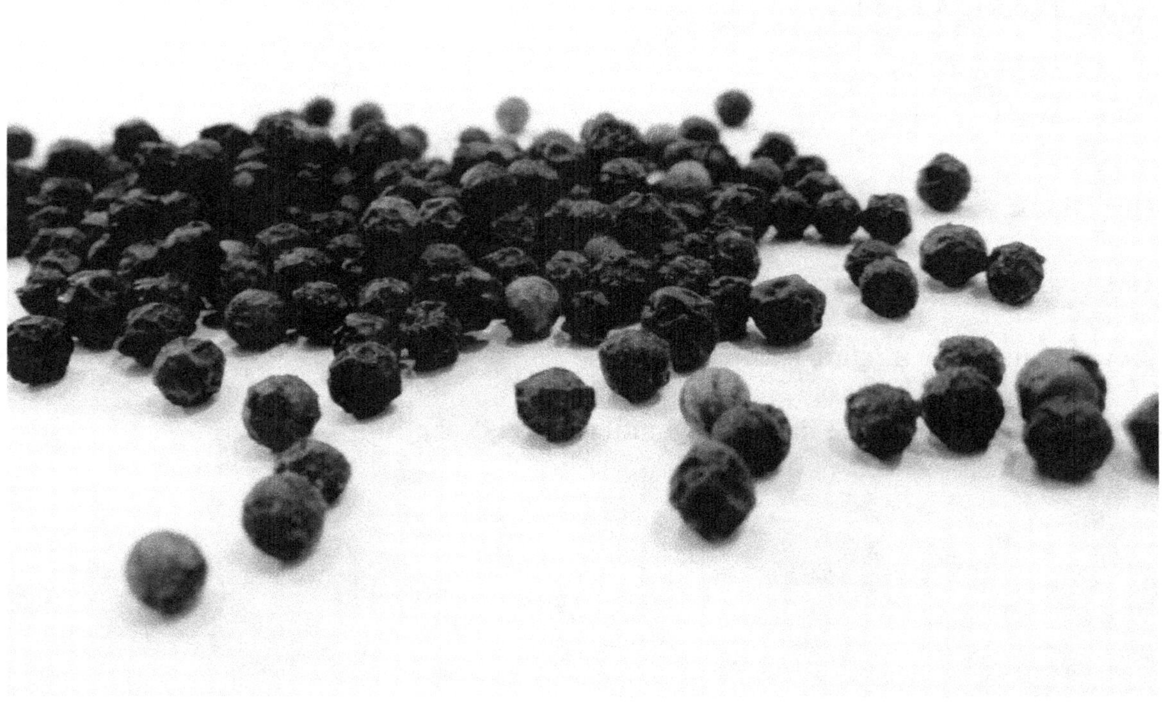

A soothing cup of tea is wonderful to drink when you are suffering from cough due to mucus buildup in the lungs. Believe it or not, the tea works as a sort of anti-inflammatory agent.

Prep Time: 10 minutes

Yields: 2 cups

Ingredients:

- Ginger, 8 slices
- Peppercorns, 1 tsp.
- Honey, 1 tsp.
- Water, 2 cups

Directions:

1. Add ginger and peppercorns to boiling water and simmer about 10 minutes.

2. Add honey after mixture is cool.

3. You can drink the tea 3 times a day until mucus is gone.

Lemon Honey and Thyme Cough Syrup Home Remedy

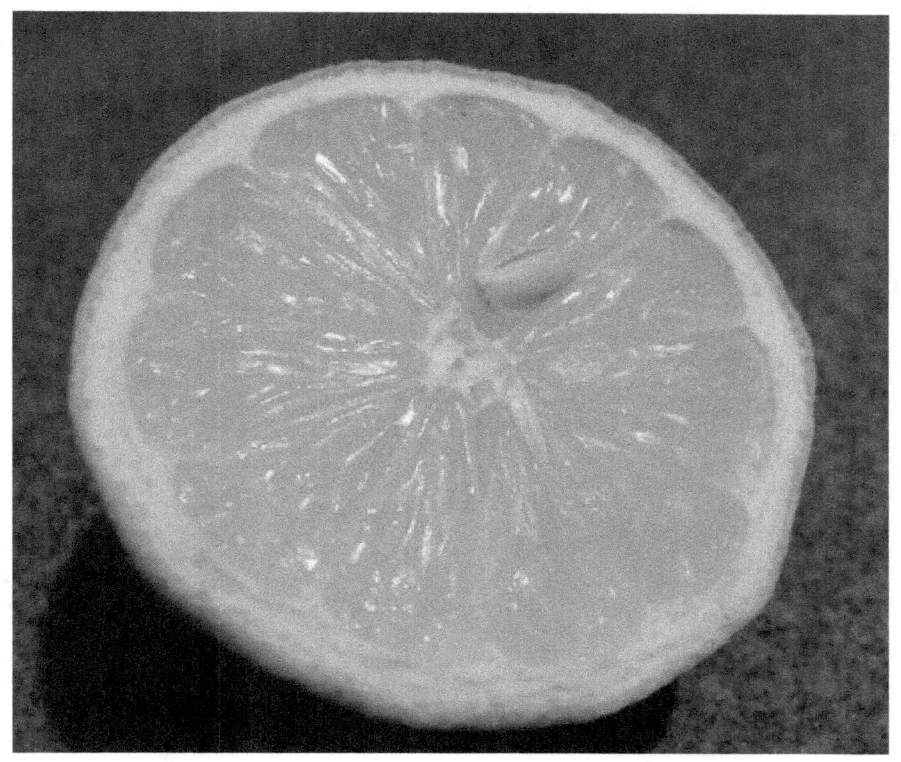

This is soothing for the cough and a sore throat. This cough syrup is wonderful for children and adults.

Prep Time: 30 minutes

Yields: 1 cup

Ingredients:

- Fresh Thyme, Several Sprigs
- Water, 2 cups
- Honey, ½ cup
- Lemon, ½ chopped

1. Combine the lemon and water and set aside for a while.

2. Simmer the thyme with water until the amount is reduced to half.

3. Strain, then add it to the jar with lemons.

4. Shake well and store until ready for use.

Honey Cinnamon Sore Throat Lollipops

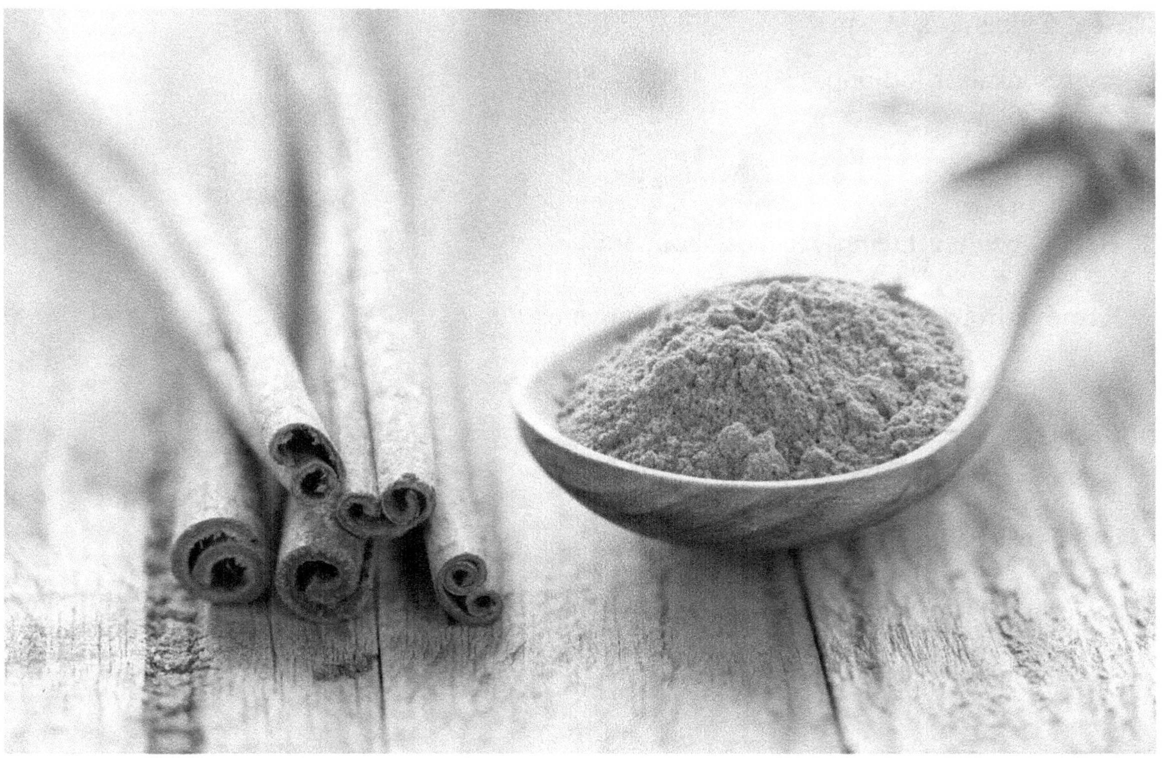

This is a great way to get the kids to take medicine. Form it into the shape of a lollipop. They will think that they are getting a treat. These lollipops are great for sore throats.

Prep Time: 10 minutes

Yields: 3 Lollipops

Ingredients:

- Honey, 1/3 cup
- Cinnamon, ¼ tsp.
- Sticks for lollipops, 3

Directions:

1. Heat honey until temp. reaches about 300'.

2. Remove from heat, let cool and add cinnamon.

3. Lay lollipop sticks on wax paper.

4. Pour mixture over top of stick, then let harden.

5. Use as needed.

Bourbon Cough Syrup Home Remedy

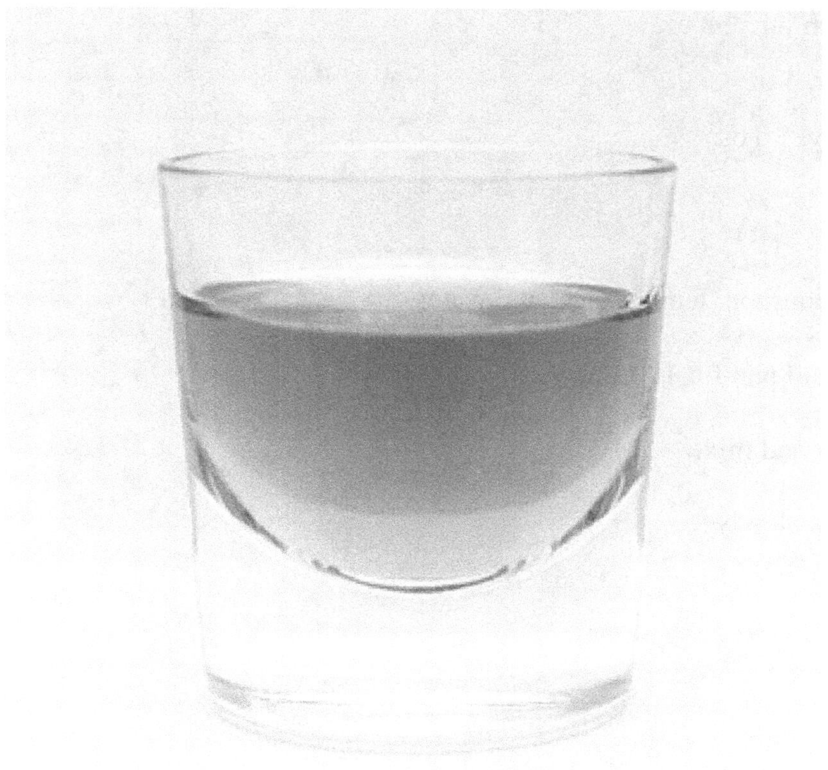

Of course, this one is for adults. This is an old recipe passed down from Grandparents. It's almost like a hot toddy.

Prep Time: 20 minutes

Yields: ½ cup

Ingredients:

- Bourbon, 2 oz.
- Lemon juice, 2 oz.
- Water, 4 oz.
- Honey, 1 Tbs.

Directions:

1. Combine bourbon, lemon juice, and water.

2. Heat in small pan for 10 minutes.

3. Add honey and mix.

4. Sip the mix slowly.

Cough Drops Homemade Recipe

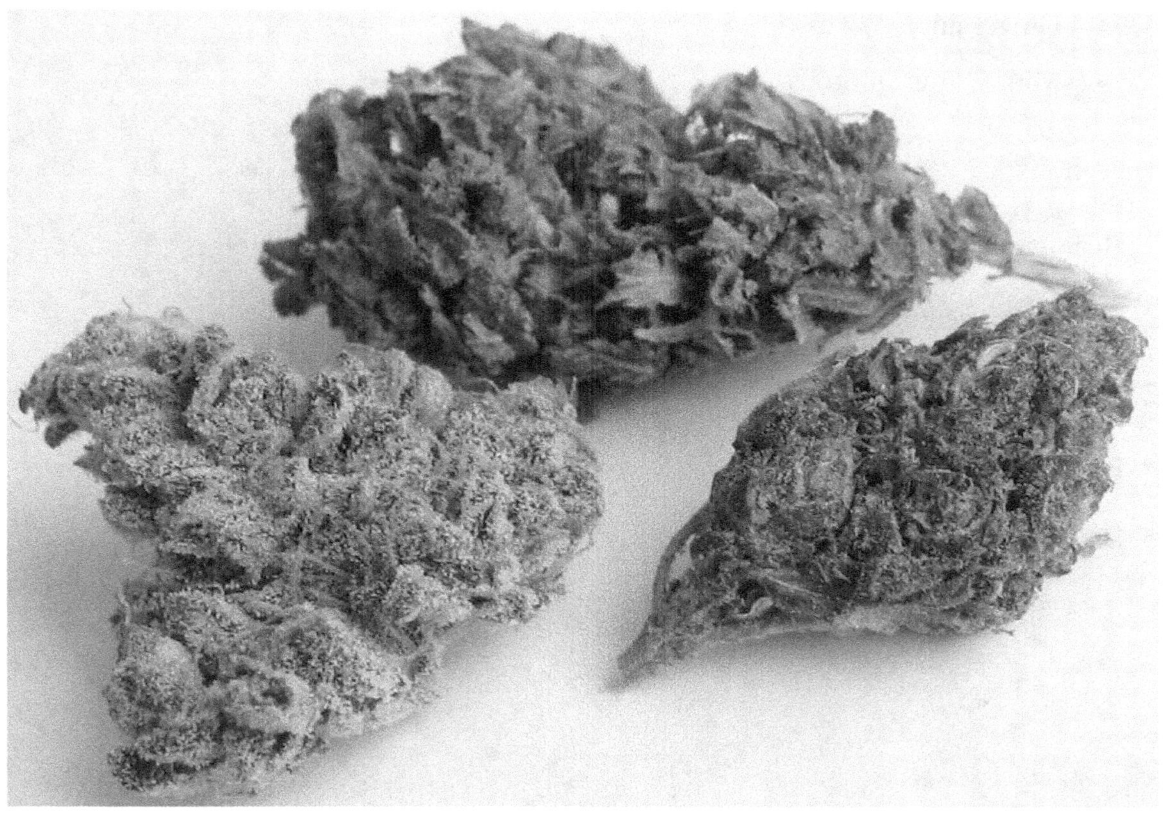

Cough drops do wonders when you are in bed or out in public. It is no fun having a coughing episode and not have anything to help to stop it. Take these with you to use when needed.

Prep Time: 30 minutes

Yields: 20 cough drops

Ingredients:

- Honey, 1 cup
- Ginger juice, ½ Tbs.
- Mint Extract, 4 drops

Directions:

1. Heat the honey until the temperature is 300'.

2. Add the ginger and mint extract when honey is ready.

3. Drop by spoonful on wax paper.

4. Let harden, then store.

5. Use when needed for cough.

Hot Toddy Homemade Recipe

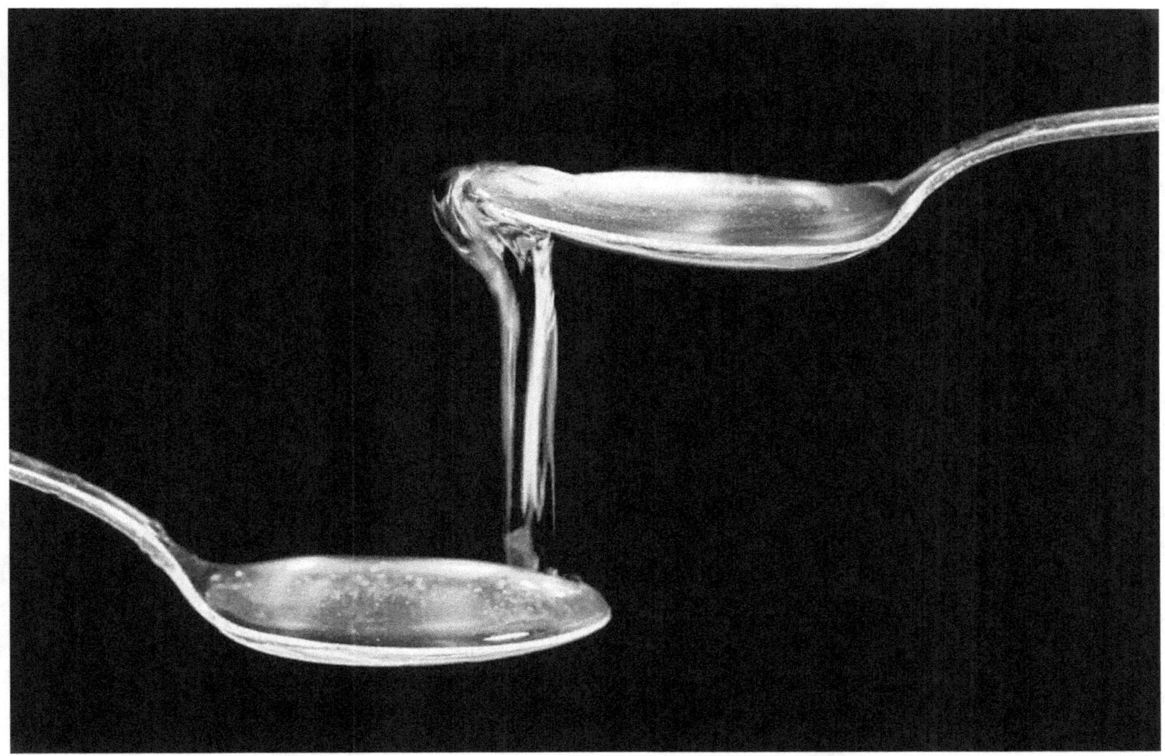

This makes a wonderful drink before bedtime or when you feel a cold coming over. It warms and relaxes the body, which helps the healing process.

Prep Time: 30 minutes

Yields: 1 Toddy

Ingredients:

- Hot Water, 1 cup
- Honey, 1 Tbs.
- Lemon, ¼
- Whole cloves, 3
- Cinnamon Stick, ½
- Brandy, 1 ½ oz.

Directions:

1. Make sure water is hot, then pour into a cup.

2. Add the honey, cloves, and cinnamon stick and mix.

3. Cool for a bit, then add the lemon and brandy.

4. Stir with the cinnamon stick, then sip until gone.

Flu Relief Homemade Recipe

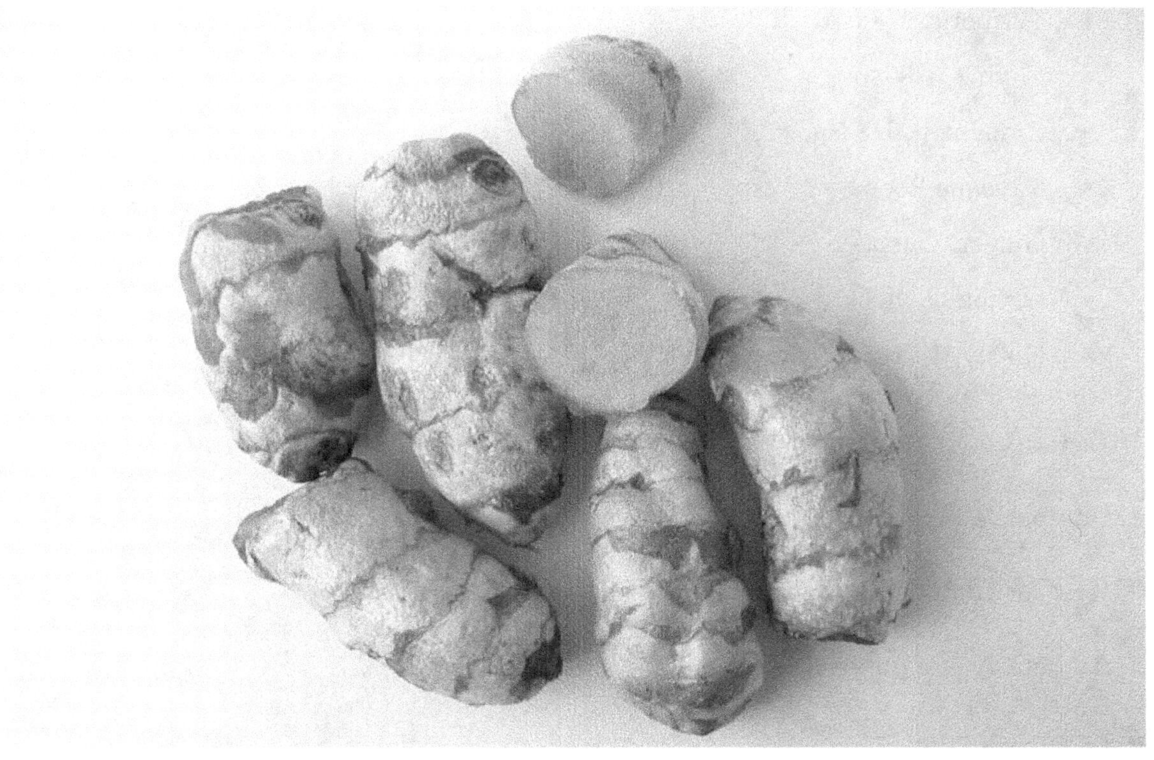

The dreaded flu season is upon us. The medicines they give to assist with the systems sometimes makes a person sick. Who wants to be sick on top of the flu. This homemade recipe is a safe one to take in order to feel some better.

Prep Time: 30 minutes

Yields: 1 cup

Ingredients:

- Water, 8 oz.
- Turmeric, 1/8 tsp.
- Thyme, 1/8 tsp
- Cinnamon, 1/8 tsp.
- Cayenne Pepper, 1/8 tsp.
- Ginger, ¼ tsp.
- Lemon, 2 slices
- Honey, 2 Tbs.

Directions:

1. Combine all ingredients except honey, in the saucepan.

2. Heat for 10 minutes, then let cool before you add the honey.

3. Add honey and mix well.

4. Enjoy feeling better.

Miscellaneous Remedies for The Entire Body

Toothache Homemade Remedy

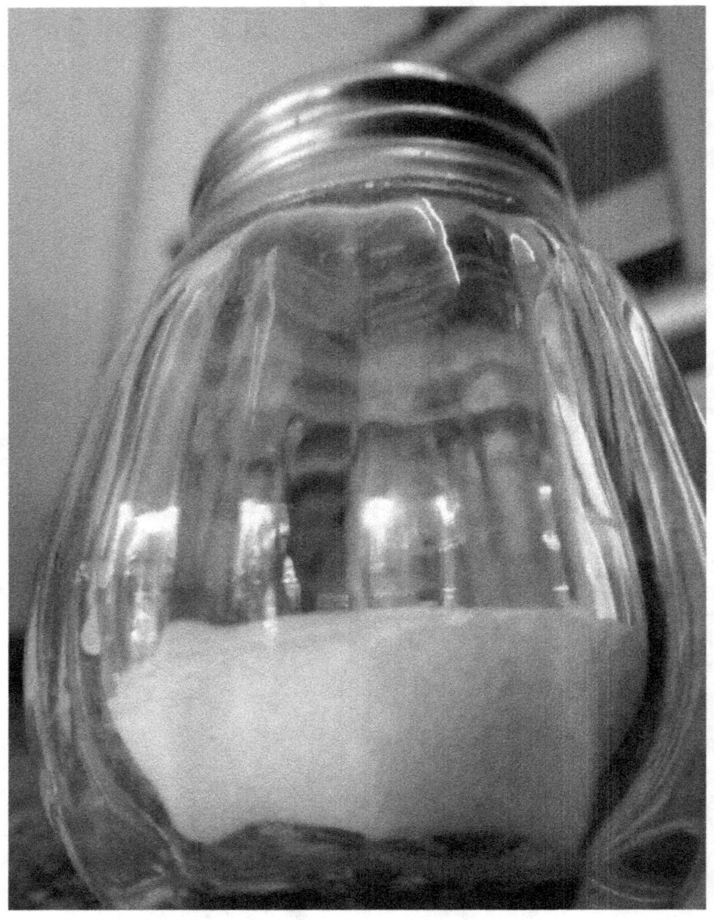

Nothing is more painful than a throbbing toothache. We have all had them. They usually hit at night when the dentist is not in. This remedy will ease the pain until you can go to the dentist.

Prep Time: 20 minutes

Yields: 1 glass

Ingredients:

- Water, 8 oz.
- Salt, ½ tsp.

Directions:

1. Combine water and salt. Mix well.

2. Swish in mouth. Then spit out.

Other suggestions:

1. Place clove oil on the affected tooth until pain diminishes.

2. You can rinse with hydrogen peroxide and water, but do not swallow.

3. Make a paste of garlic, then apply to the affected tooth.

Constipation Homemade Remedy

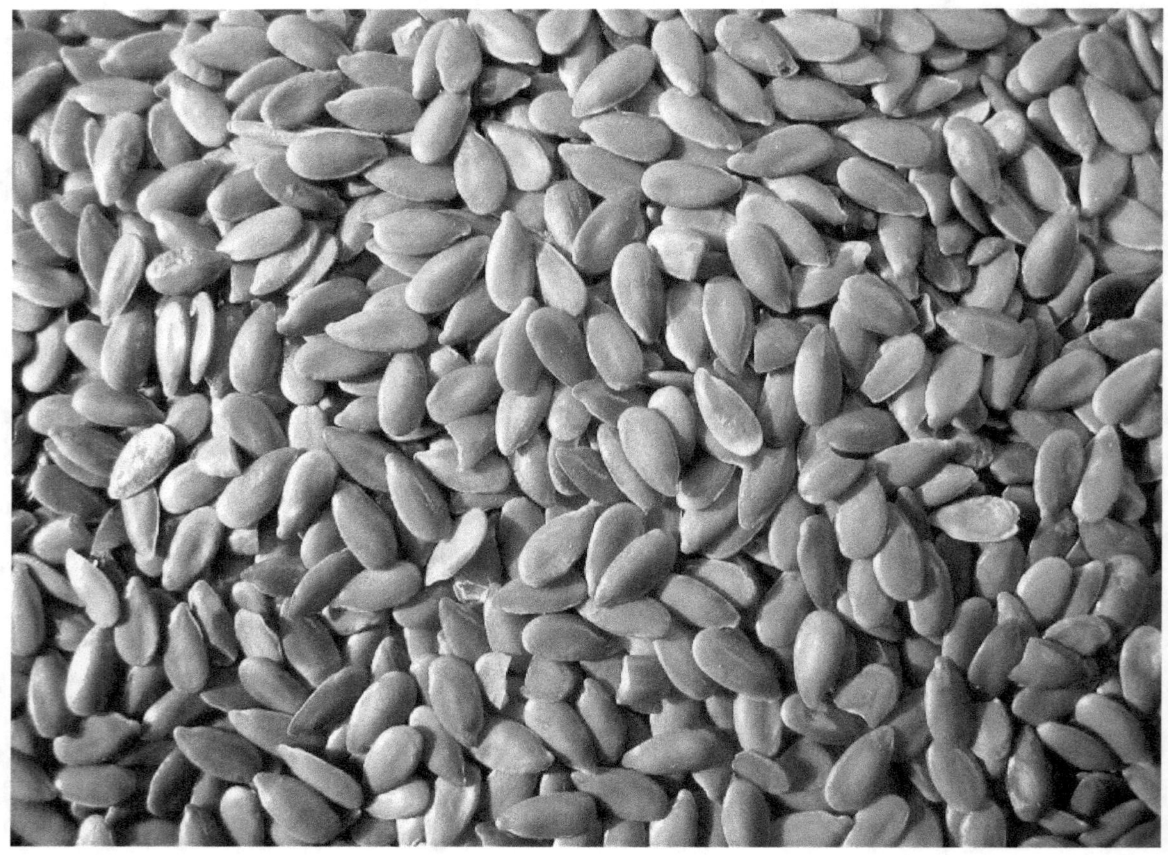

If anyone has had constipation, it is a very uncomfortable feeling, and we want relief fast. This is a sure way to help your constipation with natural ingredients.

Prep Time: 20 minutes

Yields: ½ cup

Ingredients:

- Flax Seeds, 1/4 cup
- Sunflower Seeds, 3
- Sesame Seeds, 4 to 5

Directions:

1. Grind all the seeds until you get a powdery consistency.

2. Take 1 Tablespoon daily to get constipation relief.

Eczema Home Remedy

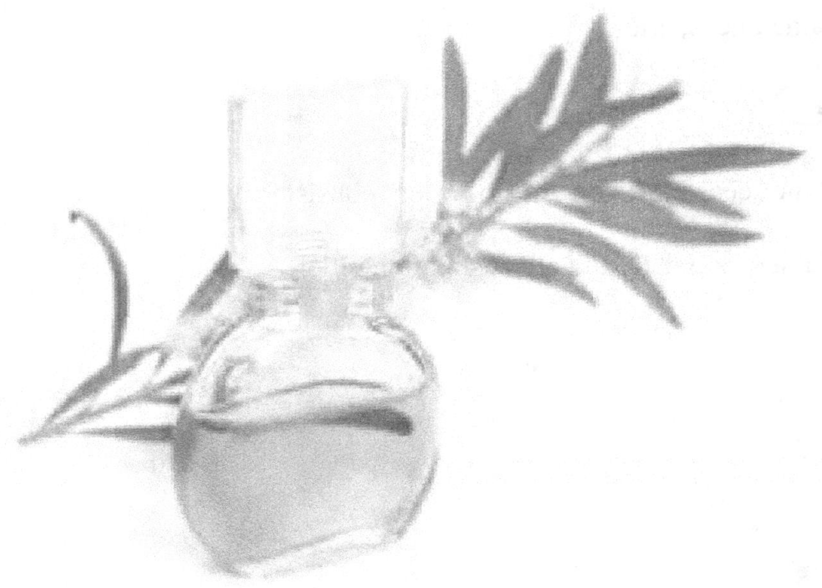

I am lucky enough not to have eczema; however, I have a close friend that has it. She worked a high-stress job, so hers flared up often. Some of the doctor's recommendations were not what she wanted, and some were painful. This one is easy on the skin and does help with the itching.

Prep Time: 10 minutes

Yields: ½ cup

Ingredients:

- Tea Tree Oil, 20 drops
- Coconut Oil, ½ cup

Directions:

1. Combine the tea tree oil and coconut oil. Mix well.

2. Rub on the affected area 2 times a day.

Bladder Infection Home Remedy

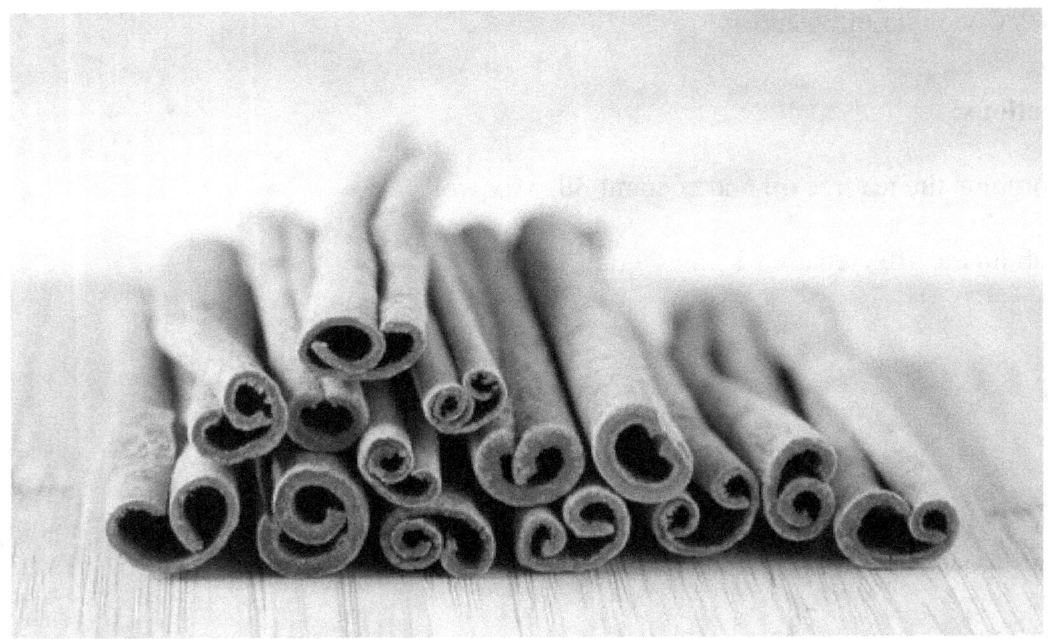

The uncomfortable feeling of bladder infection can be eased. You can take some over the counter medicine which will turn your urine orange, but this one is a simple easy mixture.

Prep Time: 10 minutes

Yields: 1 glass

Ingredients:

- Cinnamon, 2 tsp.
- Honey, 1 tsp.
- Water, 1 lukewarm

Directions:

1. Combine all ingredients together and mix well.

2. Drink this glass.

(This mixture will get rid of the germs in the bladder, which causes the infection.)

Toenail Fungus Removal Home Remedy

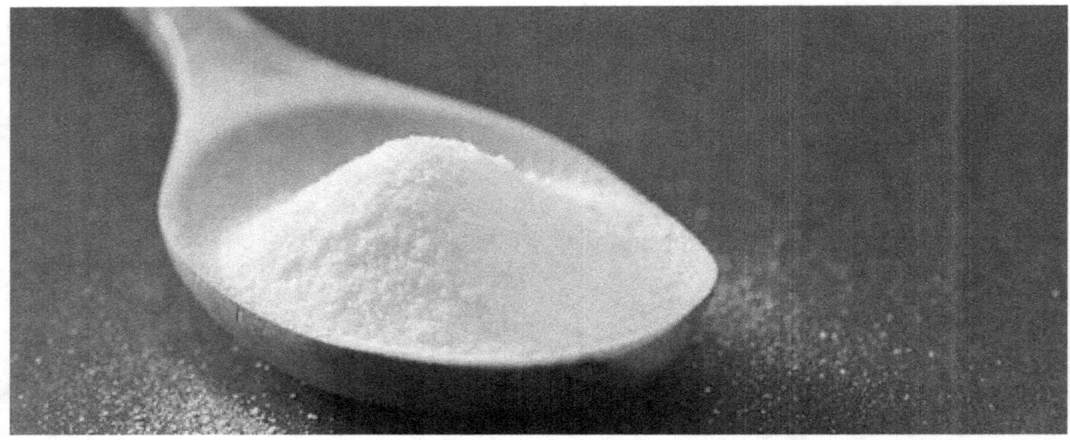

Toenail fungus is a common occurrence among people. When this is caught in time, it can be dealt with at home. This is an easy recipe to follow.

Prep Time: 10 minutes

Yields: 1-foot bath

Ingredients:

- 5 Tbs. baking soda
- 1 cup white vinegar
- Water to fill a foot tub.

Directions:

1. Combine baking soda, white vinegar and water and pour in foot bath.

2. Soak feet about 20 minutes a day.

3. Dry feet after the soak.

4. You can do this two times a day for a couple of weeks until fungus is gone.

Blood Pressure Lowering Home Remedy

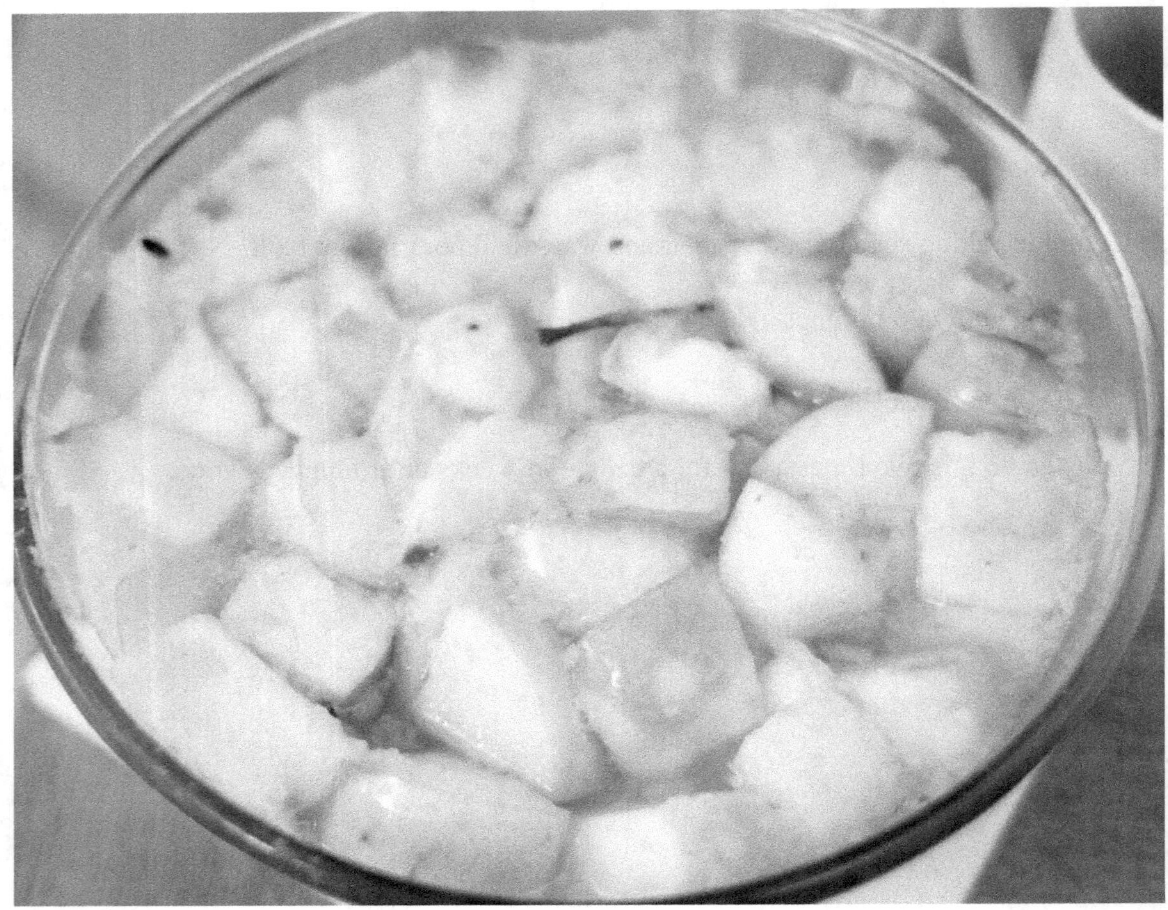

I suffer from high blood pressure and take two pills a day. I would like to try this natural remedy to see if it helps. This is to be done with a doctor's permission.

Prep Time: 10 minutes

Yields: 1 glass

Ingredients:

- Apple Cider Vinegar, 1 Tbs.
- Baking Soda, 1/8 tsp.

Directions:

1. Combine the above ingredients and mix well.

2. Drink this mixture twice daily.

(You can also drink lemon in water and drink it daily.)

High Cholesterol Home Remedy

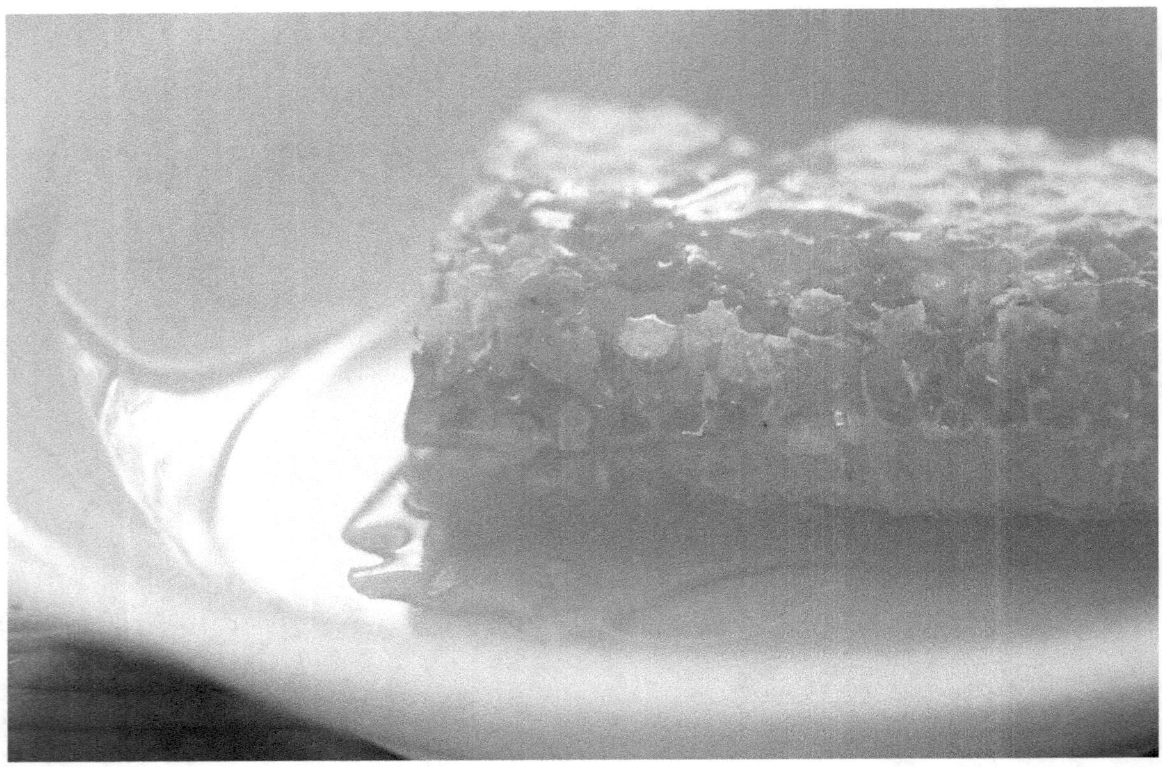

I also have high cholesterol. I take a pill at night and watch my diet, but I have read that statins can cause memory loss over a long period of time. If this works, I am ready.

Prep Time: 10 minutes

Yields: 1 glass

Ingredients:

- Honey, 1 tsp.
- Water, 1 glass

1. Stir into glass and combine.

2. Drink 1 glass daily.

(This is a cholesterol lowering ingredient. You can also use apple cider vinegar or drink a glass of orange juice daily.)

Burn Salve Home Remedy

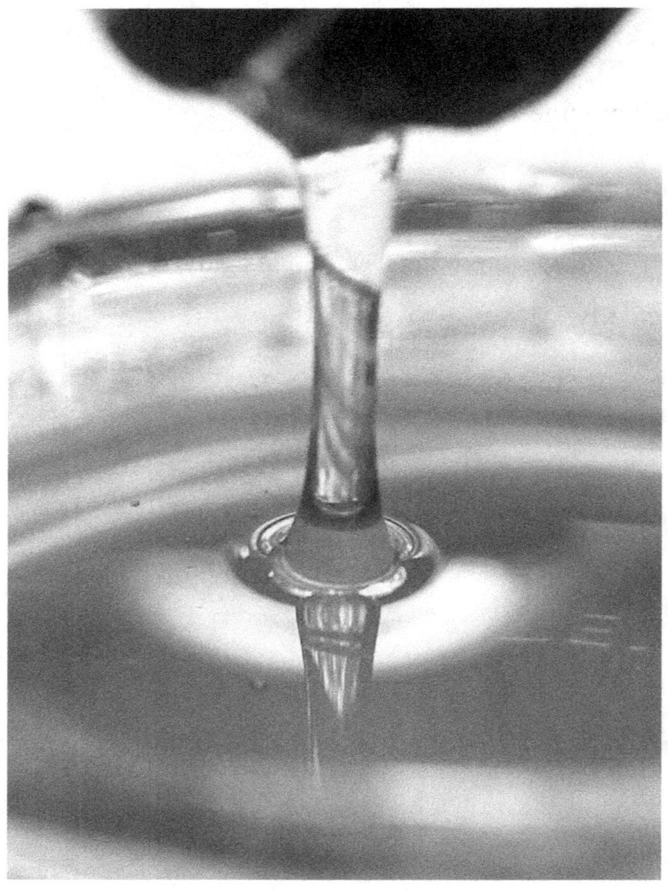

A burn can consist of a burn from a stove or sunburn. There are several kinds of burns and at different degrees. The minor ones can be eased with this soothing salve. More severe burns should be treated by a physician.

Prep Time: 30 minutes

Yields: 1 small jar

Ingredients:

- Raw honey, ¼ cup
- Coconut Oil, ¼ cup
- Beeswax, 1 tsp.
- Sea Buckthorn Oil, 1 Tbs.
- Aloe Vera Gel, ½ tsp.

Directions:

1. Heat the beeswax on stove until melted.

2. Add the coconut oil and mix together.

3. Combine the honey, aloe vera gel and Sea Buckthorn Oil with the beeswax mixture.

4. Pour into jar or tin and let set until hardened.

5. It will be able to use once hardened.

Home Cleaning Remedies

Fake Bleach Home Remedy

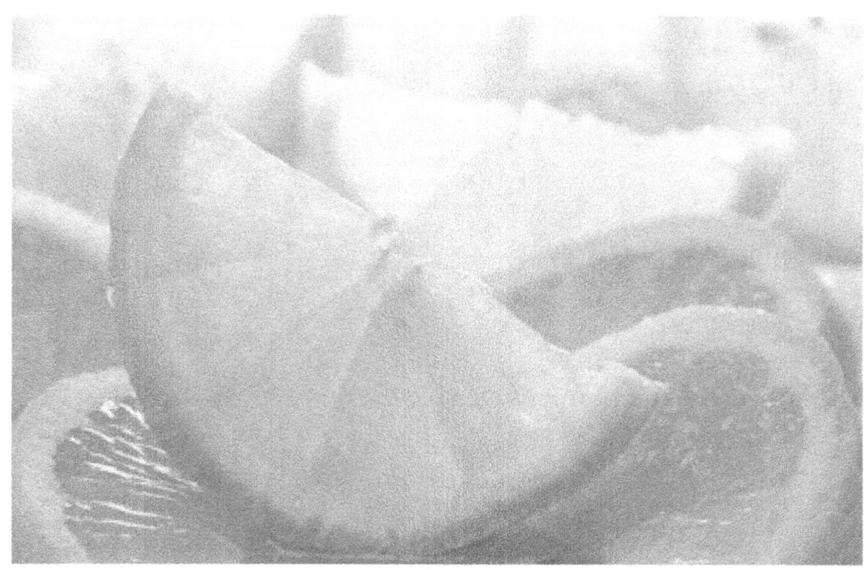

I admit that I love the smell of bleach. To me, it is a clean smell. I do use bleach a lot in cleaning, especially in the bathroom and in my white clothes. This, however, does not smell like bleach but smell like a nice lemon.

Prep Time: 10 minutes

Yields: 1 spray bottle full

Ingredients:

- Hydrogen Peroxide, 1 cup
- Water, 1 cup
- Lemon Oil, 20 drops

Directions:

1. Combine all of the above ingredients.

2. Pour into spray bottle and shake.

3. Use on anything you would normally use bleach on.

Carpet Cleaner Homemade Recipe

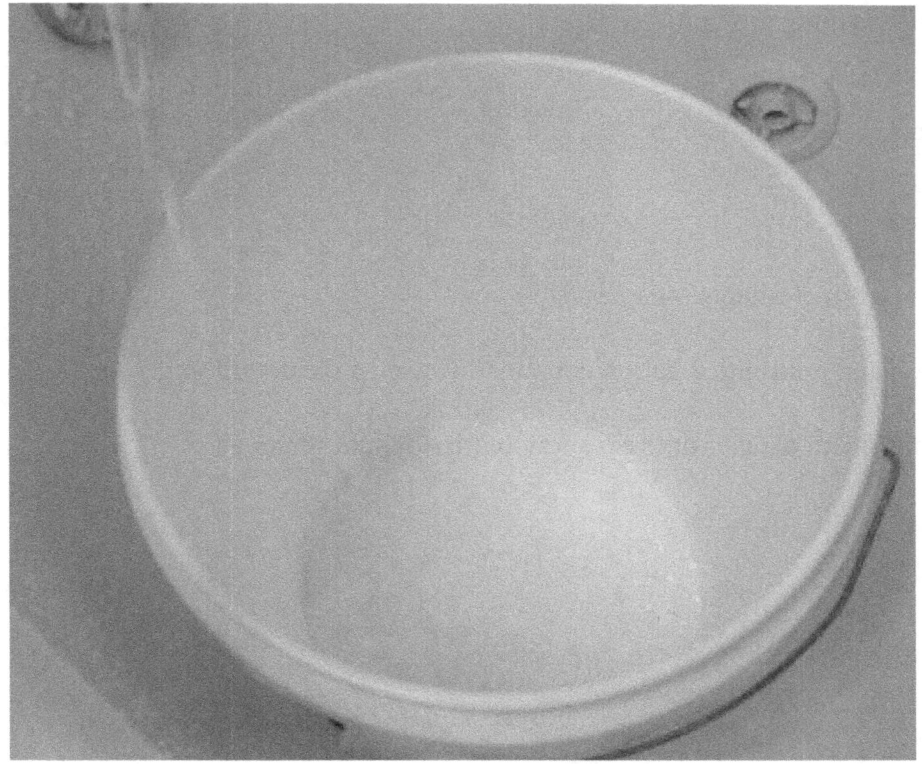

I made this recipe and used it in one of the rental steam cleaners. It was great. Not only did it get my carpet clean, but it was much cheaper than if I had to buy carpet cleaner to put into the machine. I highly recommend the cleaner.

Prep Time: 10 minutes

Yields: Several gallons

Ingredients:

- Hydrogen Peroxide, 1 cup
- Dish Liquid, 1/8 cup
- Oxiclean, 1 Tbs.
- Fabric Softener, ½ cup

Directions:

1. Combine all ingredients together.

2. Mix well and pour into a gallon container. (I used a clean milk jug.)

3. Pour into steam cleaner or use a spray bottle for spot removal.

Homemade Fabric Softner Recipe

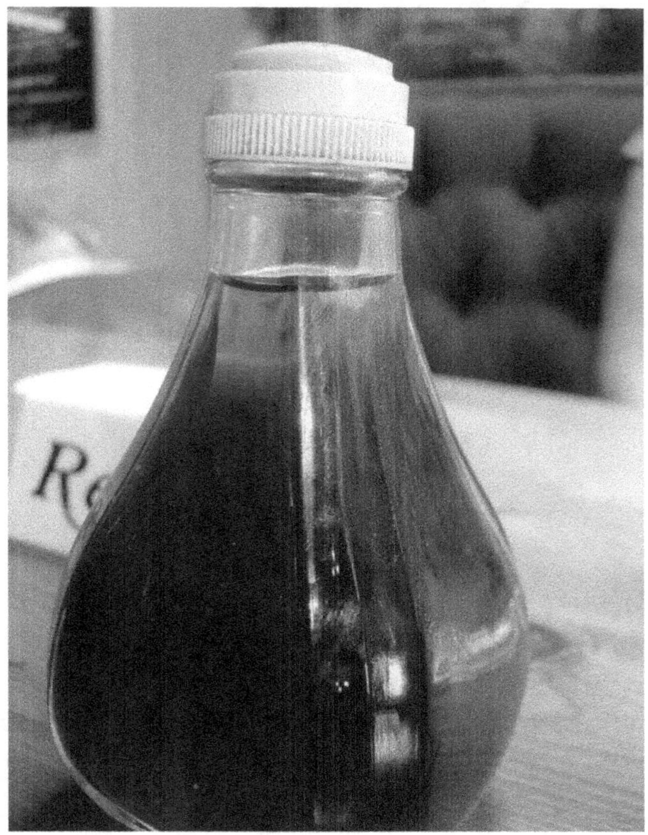

I admit that I use dryer sheets most of the time because of convenience. However, I do like the liquid fabric softener's smell. I use it most of the time on whites and towels. They smell fresher.

Prep Time: 15 minutes

Yields: 3 cups

Ingredients:

- Hot water, 3 cups
- Vinegar, 1 ½ cup
- Hair Conditioner, 1 cup

Directions:

1. Combine conditioner and vinegar with the hot water.

2. Pour into a container and shake.

3. Use as you would use your normal fabric softener.

Homemade Clorox Wipes

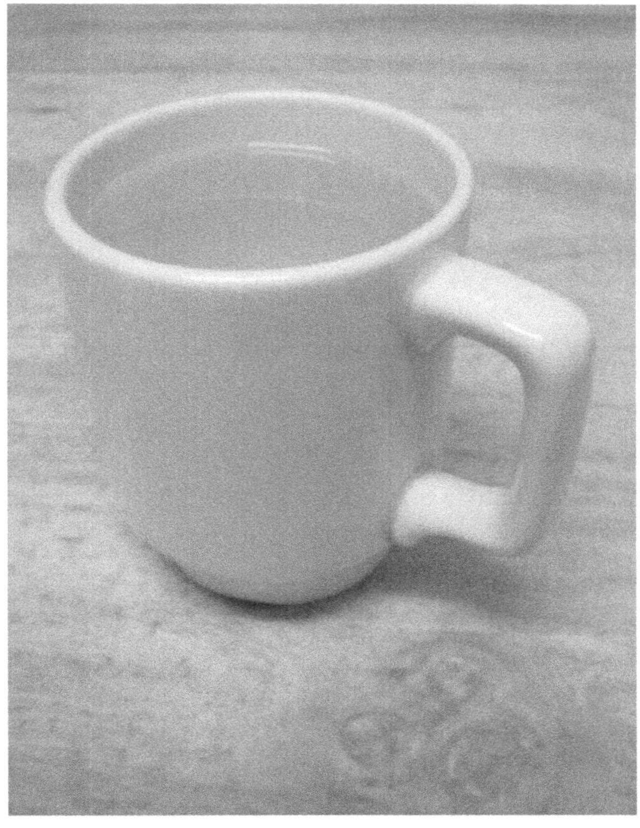

These come in very handy for spills and small cleaning jobs. I like to keep this in my kitchen, especially when I am cooking. At that time, it is easy to make a lot of small messes.

Prep Time: 10 minutes

Yields: 1 container

Ingredients:

- Water, 1 cup
- Alcohol, ¼ cup
- Dawn Dish Soap, 2 Tbs.
- Ammonia, 2 Tbs.
- Paper towel Roll, cut in 1/4

Directions:

1. Place the paper towel roll in container where you can pull up through the pull out

2. Combine all the ingredients above.

3. Pour over paper towels and close top.

4. Dispose of paper towels when you use them.

Dishwasher Detergent Home Recipe

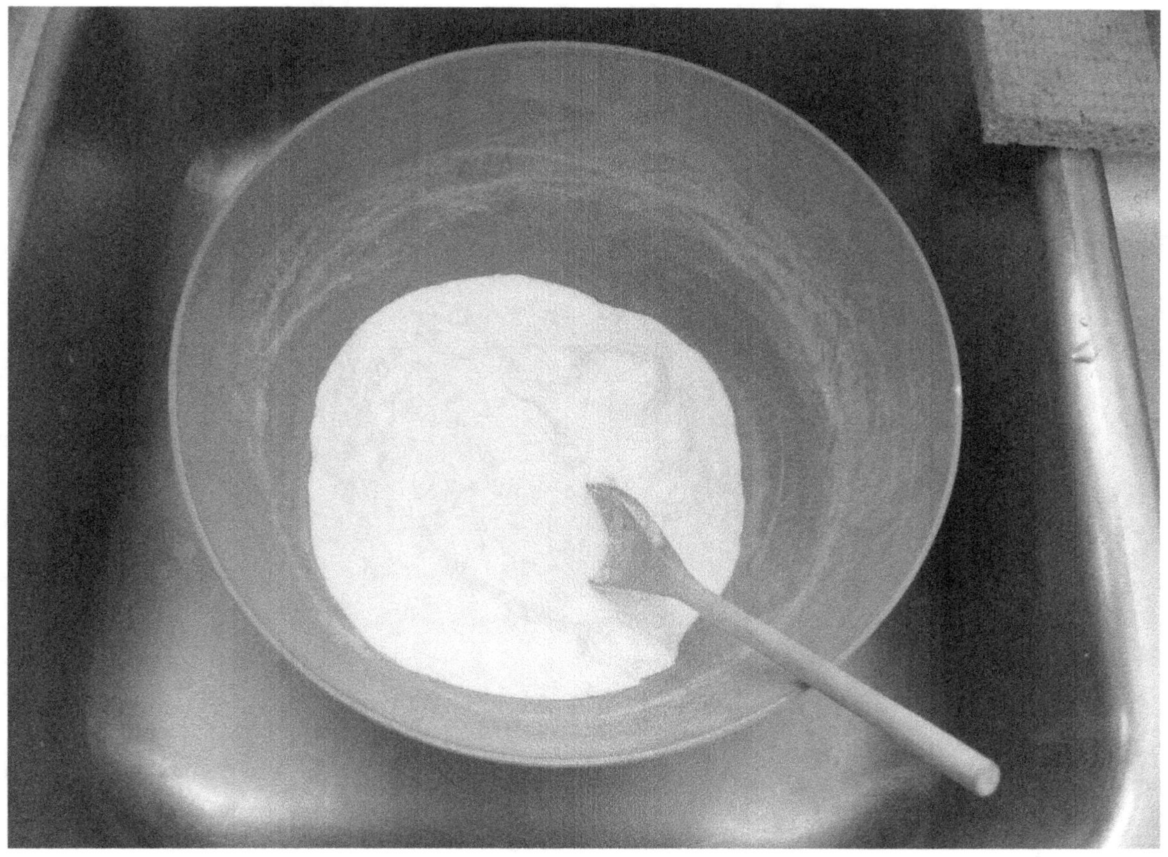

I hate to run out of dishwasher detergent. This recipe is very helpful when that happens. I can make up a small batch and continue washing my dishes.

Prep Time: 10 minutes

Yields: 1 cup

Ingredients:

- Baking Soda, 1 cup
- Borax, 1 cup
- Scented Oil, 2 drops

Directions:

1. Combine the above ingredients and store.

2. Use as you would normally use the store-bought dishwasher detergent.

Homemade Dusting Spray Recipe

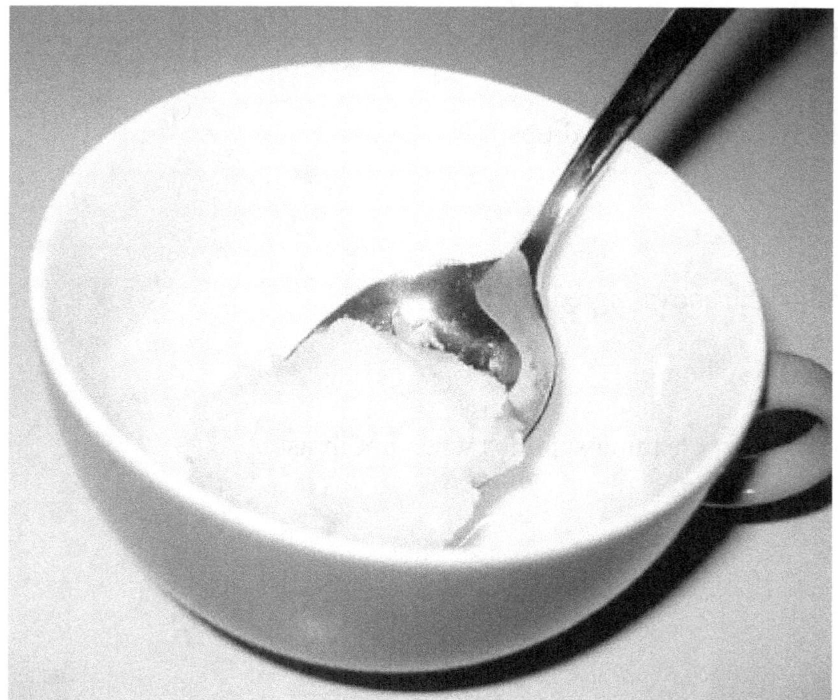

I love my room to smell good. Usually, the dusting spray used reflects this. It can be costly at the store, but this quick recipe does a great job.

Prep Time: 10 minutes

Yields: 1 spray bottle, 16 0z.

Ingredients:

- Distilled Water, 1 cup
- White Vinegar, ½ cup
- Coconut Oil, ¼ cup
- Orange Essential Oil, 30 drops

Directions:

1. Combine all of the above ingredients.

2. Pour into the spray bottle.

3. Store with the other cleaning supplies when not in use.

Homemade Glass Cleaner Recipe

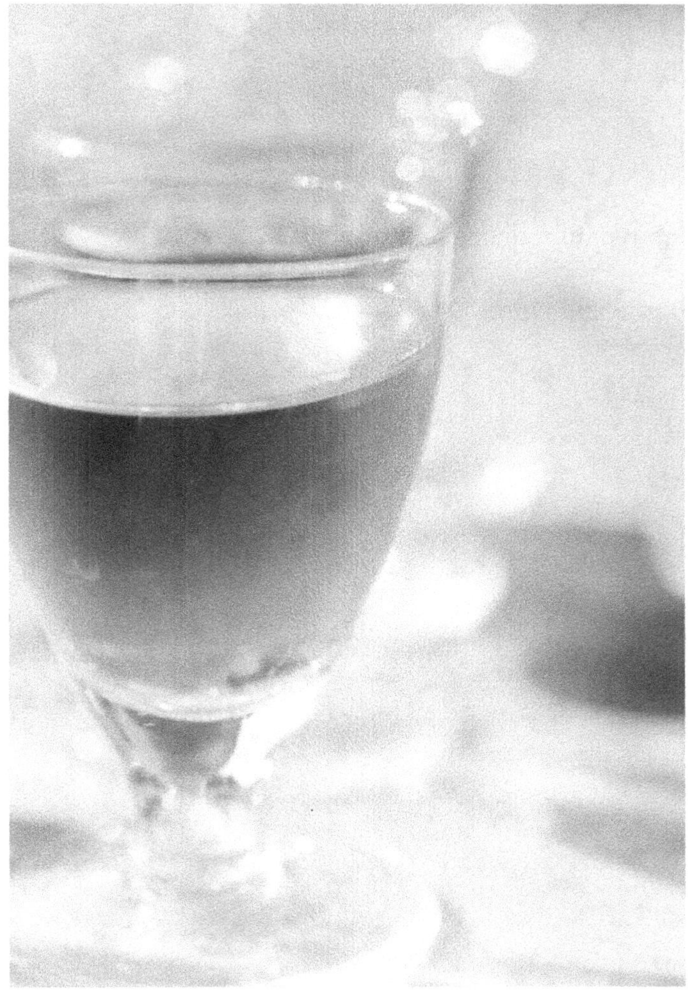

Glass cleaner is important to me. I do not like the ones that streak. Using vinegar in this one helps with no streaking. I always use straight vinegar and water to clean windows.

Prep Time: 10 minutes

Yields: Small Spray Bottle

Ingredients:

- Water, 1 cup
- Alcohol, 1 cup
- Vinegar, 1 Tbs.

Directions:

1. Combine all the above ingredients and mix well.

2. Pour into spray bottle and store.

Homemade Laundry Detergent Recipe

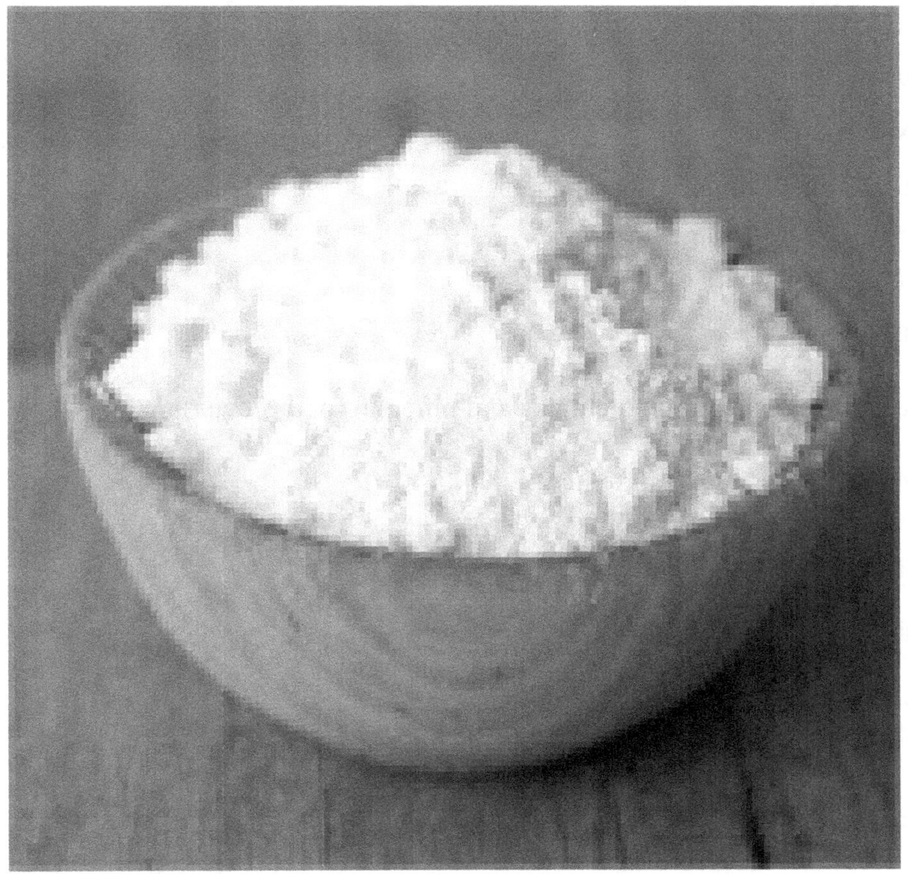

Everyone knows that detergents are a high price. This recipe will be cheaper and makes more than you get at the store. It will save you money and smells great.

Prep Time: 10 minutes

Yields: 2 gallons

Ingredients:

- Arm & Hammer Washing Soap, 55 oz.
- Baking Soda, 4 lb. box
- Borax, 76 oz.
- Oxi Clean, 3 lb.
- Fels Naptha Laundry Soap, 4 bars
- Washer Enhancer Beads, 13,2 oz.

Directions:

1. First, cut the Fels Naptha into chunks and puree in food processor.

2. Use a garbage can to mix ingredients.

3. Empty all ingredients into garbage can, close and mix well.

4. Pour into the 2-gallon container.

5. Use 2 -3 Tbs. for each load of clothes.

Homemade Toilet Bomb Recipe

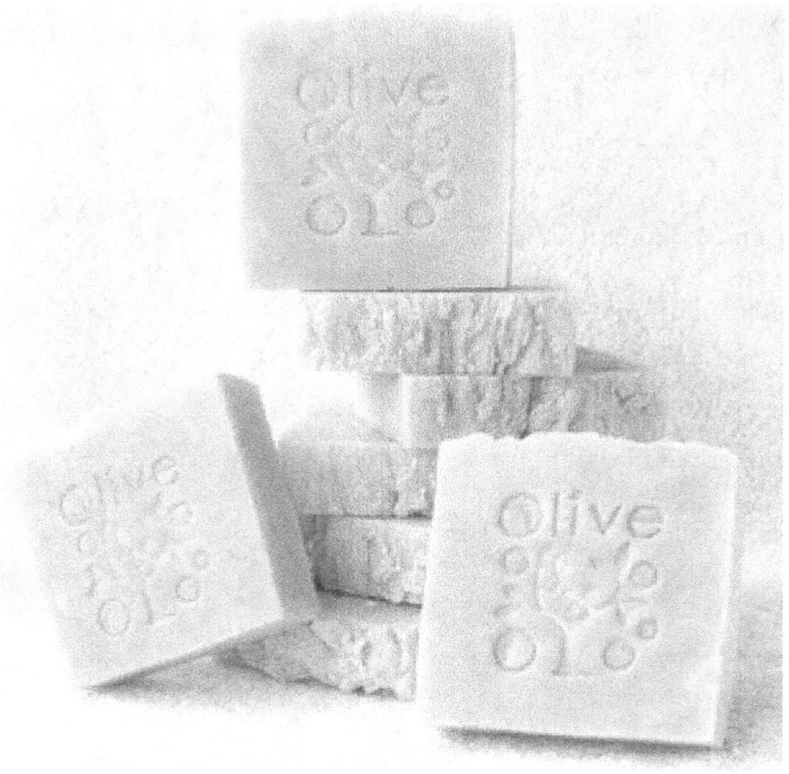

Toilet cleaning is not a favorite chore for anyone. These homemade bombs help to keep your toilet fresh and clean in between cleanings. That way, you don't need to clean it every week anymore.

Prep Time: 10 minutes

Yields: 12

Ingredients:

- Baking Soda, 1 cup
- Citric Acid, ¼ cup
- Castile Soap, 1 ½ tsp.

Directions:

1. Combine the above ingredients.

2. Form into balls and fit into mold.

3. Let the toilet bombs sit overnight.

4. Store in container with lid until use.

5. Keep in bathroom closet and drop 1 in.

Room Deodorizer Spray Recipe

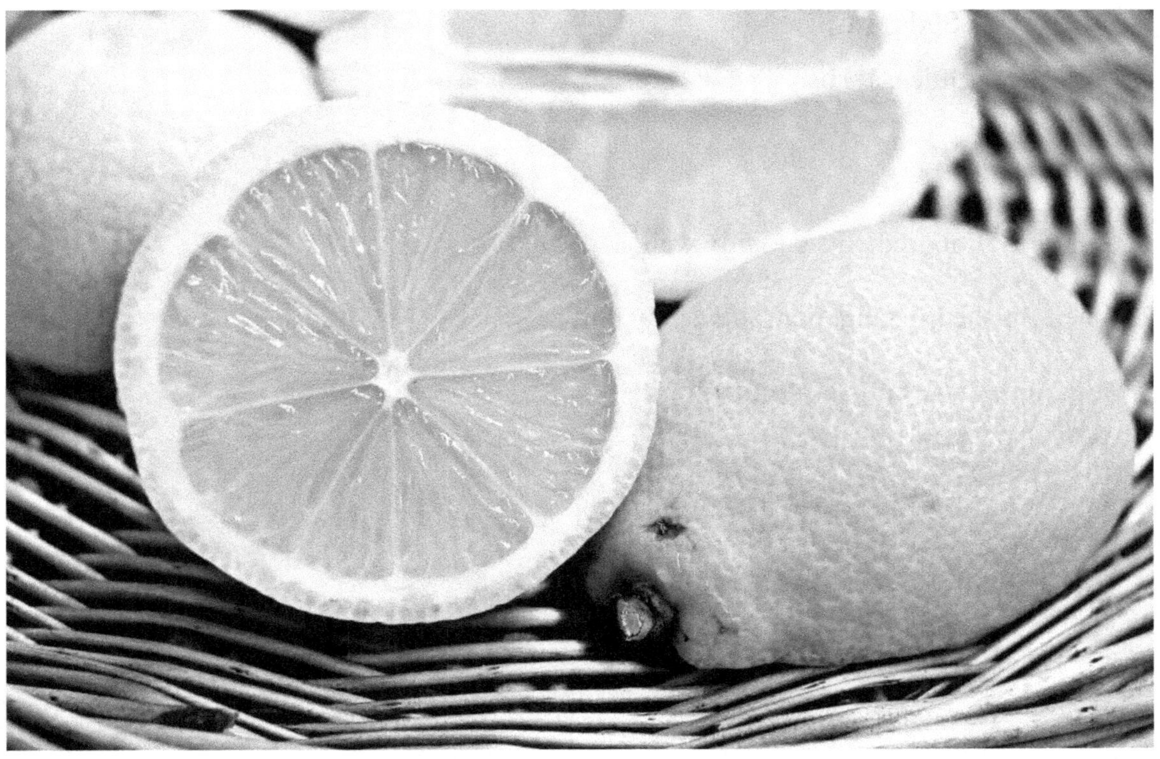

Hey, everyone has a stinky room now and then. Whether it be from pets or children, the odors can be overwhelming. This deodorizer spray works great to eliminate the bad smells.

Prep Time: 10 minutes

Yields: 1 spray bottle

Ingredients:

- Distilled Water, 1 ¾ cups
- Baking Soda, 1 tsp
- Lemon Juice, 1 Tbs.

Directions:

1. Combine all ingredients and mix well.

2. When finished fizzing, pour into spray bottle.

3. Begin spraying, safe on furniture.

Author's Afterthoughts

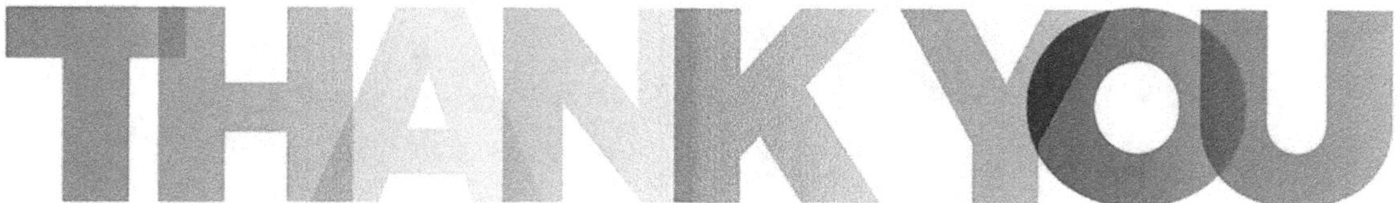

Thanks ever so much to each of my cherished readers for investing the time to read this book!

I know you could have picked from many other books, but you chose this one. So, a big thanks for downloading this book and reading all the way to the end.

If you enjoyed this book or received value from it, I'd like to ask you for a favor. Please take a few minutes to post an honest and heartfelt review on Amazon.com. Your support does make a difference and helps to benefit other people.

Thanks for your Reviews!

Rachael Rayner